Dr Atkins
Diet
PLANNER

Other publications by
Dr Robert C Atkins available from Vermilion

Dr Atkins New Diet Revolution
Dr Atkins New Diet Cookbook
Dr Atkins New Carbohydrate Counter
Dr Atkins Age-Defying Diet Revolution

The world's most
successful diet

Dr Atkins
Diet
PLANNER

Keep track of your weight loss
with this unique carb companion

Dr Robert C Atkins

✔ermilion

5 7 9 10 8 6 4

Copyright © 2003 by Robert C. Atkins, M.D.

First published in the United States in 2003 by M. Evans and Company, Inc.

This edition first published in the United Kingdom in 2003 by Vermilion, an imprint of Ebury Press, Random House, 20 Vauxhall Bridge Road, London SW1V 2SA
www.randomhouse.co.uk

Random House Australia (Pty) Limited
20 Alfred Street, Milsons Point, Sydney, New South Wales 2061, Australia

Random House New Zealand Limited, 18 Poland Road, Glenfield, Auckland 10, New Zealand

Random House South Africa (Pty) Limited, Endulini, 5a Jubilee Road, Parktown 2193, South Africa

The Random House Group Limited Reg. No. 954009

Papers used by Vermilion are natural, recyclable products made from wood grown in sustainable forests.

Printed and bound in Great Britain by Bookmarque Ltd, Croydon, Surrey

A CIP catalogue for this book is available from the British Library

ISBN 0091898773

Contents

```
┌─────────────────────────┐
│                         │
│                         │
│                         │
│                         │
│     PLACE YOUR          │
│     PHOTO HERE          │
│                         │
│                         │
│                         │
│                         │
│                         │
└─────────────────────────┘
```

This is me before I started doing Atkins

Why Keep a Diet Planner?

Whether you'd like to lose weight, maintain a healthy weight, or simply reduce your consumption of such empty carbohydrates as sugar and white flour, keeping a diet planner can be an invaluable ally in helping you reach your goals. The *Dr Atkins Diet Planner* is specifically designed to help you successfully comply with the low carbohydrate lifestyle outlined in *Dr Atkins New Diet Revolution*. Not only will you chart what you eat from day to day, you'll also examine your progress in several ways. That way you can track your success, as well as retrace your steps when you've temporarily gone astray (and let's face it: we all make mistakes!). It will also help you see if certain foods are getting in the way of your journey to a slimmer, healthier you. You'll get to know your eating habits, identify nutritional stumbling blocks, and explore emotions and other lifestyle issues that may have a bearing on your relationship with food.

Use this 120-day diet planner as a way to keep your goals in focus. Why did you decide to do Atkins? What benefits do you hope to achieve? By recording your progress and your thoughts, you can revisit them when you're tempted to cheat and motivate yourself by reviewing your stated goals and your successes. Keep in mind that how you feel while doing Atkins can be just important as what you eat.

Like watching your carbohydrate intake, exercising regularly, and taking your supplements, keeping a diet planner is part of a regimen that allows you to stay in control – and with that control comes the pleasure of accomplishment. Once you've reached your goals, reread this diet planner regularly to remind yourself of your achievements and to help keep yourself on the straight and narrow. Some people find it equally useful to continue keeping a diet planner as an aid to maintaining their new weight.

In addition to the diet planner pages, we have provided additional information to make doing Atkins as easy as possible. Some of that content follows directly; the rest starts on page 217.

Getting Started:
Your Personal Evaluation

Name:

Age:

Atkins Start Date:

Starting Weight:

Starting Size:

Goal Weight:

Goal Size:

STARTING BLOOD LEVELS

Total Cholesterol:

    Triglycerides:

    HDL Cholesterol:

    LDL Cholesterol:

Blood Pressure:

Glucose:

MEASUREMENTS

Chest:

Waist:

Hips:

Upper arms:

Thighs:

When and why did you decide to start doing Atkins?

Write down the goals that you'd like to achieve on Atkins. Are you trying to lose weight? To reap other health benefits? To feel better emotionally?

If you do achieve the above goals, how will your life be different?

Before You Begin

It's time to ready your kitchen, your loved ones, and your own mind-set. These seven steps will help make doing Atkins one of the most rewarding experiences of your life.

1. **Record some vital stats** before you begin. Using a tape measure, determine the measurements of your chest, waist, hips, upper arms and thighs, and write down those numbers on page 9. When you remeasure yourself in a couple of weeks, you'll be happy you did. The more ways you have of gauging your success, the more encouraged you'll be.

2. **Come up with an exercise plan.** If you aren't already exercising, start doing so now. Even a half hour of brisk walking four times a week will make a big difference, especially if you are almost completely inactive now. Exercise is a critical element of the healthy new you and will speed your weight loss. You may not want to implement this plan, however, until after the first two days on Atkins. In that 48-hour period you may feel tired and a bit off-kilter as your body makes its conversion from burning glucose to burning fat as its primary fuel. Be sure to check with your doctor before starting to exercise if you have been inactive or are stepping up your activity level.

3. **Stock the kitchen** with the food you're going to eat, including plenty of your favourite protein goodies. (See Acceptable Foods specified for the Induction phase, starting on page 23.) If you love, say, hard-boiled eggs, turkey, chicken, prawn salad, and cheese, have all these foods and more readily accessible in your refrigerator, along with plenty of salad ingredients and other vegetables low in carbs. It's crucial that you not find yourself running out of the right foods and tempted by the wrong ones when hunger strikes. You'll also want to stock up on the wide variety of low carbohydrate products available in your local health-food store or most supermarkets.

4. **Get rid of high carb foods.** That includes beverages as well as foods. This is easiest if you live alone and needn't worry about what anyone else wants in the refrigerator. Invite friends over to finish off the ice cream. Have a 'carb blowout' party. Give away all your forbidden foods, perhaps to a shelter for the homeless. As a last resort, just throw them out. Alter your mental picture: for you, these foods no longer exist.

5. **Purchase nutritional supplements** recommended for the programme so you have a good supply on hand. They are a key part of doing Atkins.

6. **Get your loved ones on your team.** Prepare the people you live with by explaining your new eating style. You will be eating many of the things you've always eaten, but passing up others full of empty carbohydrates. If you are the chief cook and bottle washer, unless you can convince the other members of your household to share the Atkins experience with you, you'll simply have to cook for yourself and prepare a few additions for them. If they want bread, potatoes and dessert, you may have to suffer a little temptation, but if you really want to lose weight you'll bite the bullet and not the breadstick.

7. **Find an Atkins buddy.** It is often easier to try something new if you have a partner to share your experience with. A friend or coworker will support your efforts and vice versa. If you don't have a weight-loss buddy, be sure to go to www.atkins.com and use 'My Atkins' for tips and other supportive information to help reinforce your efforts to create a healthier life for yourself.

See Your Doctor Before Starting the Atkins Nutritional Approach

You are probably raring to start Atkins and begin your weight-loss journey. But first, a crucial warning: people with severe kidney disease (creatinine level of over 2.4) should not do any phase of Atkins unless ordered to do so by their doctor. Also, pregnant women and nursing mothers may follow the Lifetime Maintenance phase but should not follow any of the weight-loss phases of Atkins.

If none of the above conditions apply, the first thing you should do is review any medications you are taking and make a doctor's appointment to get a complete physical, including blood checks to test your lipid levels and other tests. It's important to have a medical workup before beginning Atkins, both from a health perspective and to help motivate you to follow the programme faithfully. A physical may uncover a health problem, such as hyperinsulinism, that you were not aware of that may make doing Atkins all the more imperative. You also want to have benchmarks in addition to weight and centimetres/inches lost against which to measure your progress.

With that in mind, let's look at the medical steps you should take before you begin to change your eating habits. You should stop taking any nonessential over-the-counter medications, such as cough syrup or cough drops, antacids, sleep aids, antihistamines or laxatives. Many prescription medications also inhibit weight loss. Talk to your doctor to see if an alternative can be found. There are also several categories of drugs that can cause adverse effects when taken while on a low carbohydrate eating plan. First are the diuretics, because reducing your carbohydrate intake alone can have a dramatic diuretic effect. Secondly, since Atkins is so effective at lowering high blood sugar, people who take insulin or oral diabetes medications that stimulate insulin can end up with dangerously low blood-sugar levels. Thirdly, Atkins has a strong blood pressure–lowering effect and can easily convert blood pressure medications into an overdose. If you are currently taking any of these medications, you will need your doctor's help to adjust your dosages.

Be sure your doctor measures your blood chemistries and lipid levels (write the results down on page 9) – and quite possibly administers a glucose-tolerance test, with insulin levels drawn at fasting and at one- and two-hour intervals – before you start the programme. Lipid levels will reveal your total cholesterol, HDL and LDL cholesterol, and triglycerides. These indicators often change with drastic dietary intervention. The blood chemistries will measure baseline glucose (blood sugar) as well as kidney and liver function. Be sure your doctor also measures your uric acid levels. Since some people wrongly believe these indicators are negatively affected by doing Atkins, you may later regret not having a 'before' baseline to compare with your 'after' results.

If you choose to keep track of those hidden physical changes that are measured in your blood, you'll find that after you start Atkins they should begin improving steadily. Don't wait to have your initial lab work done until after you start Atkins, because then you may think any abnormalities are the result of your new way of eating. You may well have had even higher cholesterol and triglycerides before you began.

Your doctor will also check your blood pressure. High blood pressure – known as 'the silent killer' – and being overweight often go together. High blood pressure (also called hypertension) puts you at clear risk for stroke and heart disease and may indicate elevated insulin levels. What happens to high blood pressure on Atkins? It goes down. Nothing is more consistently or more rapidly observed than normalization of blood pressure.

What Is the Atkins Nutritional Approach?

The cornerstone of the Atkins philosophy is a four-phase eating plan in conjunction with vitamin and mineral supplementation and regular exercise. The Atkins Nutritional Approach is a safe, effective way to lose weight steadily and easily. But even more importantly, it allows you to achieve your goal weight – permanently. Understanding the four phases of doing Atkins is crucial to your success. Here's a quick summary of how they work:

Phase 1: Induction. To get your weight-loss programme off to a fast start, you limit your carbohydrate intake to just 20 g of Net Carbs a day for a minimum of two weeks. (Net Carbs are the only carbs that have a noted impact on blood sugar. See page 20 for more on Net Carbs.) During this time, you satisfy your appetite with foods high in protein and good fats, such as olive oil, along with three small handfuls of salad greens (dressed with your favourite low carb dressing) or two small handfuls of salad and two tablespoons of raw, non-starchy veggies such as broccoli florets or courgettes. After two weeks, you can add 25 g/1 oz of nuts or seeds to your daily intake if they don't interfere with weight loss.

Phase 2: Ongoing Weight Loss (OWL). During OWL, you continue to eat high-quality protein and fat, along with your salad greens and vegetables. Week by week, you add back nutrient-rich carbohydrates such as more veggies, cheese, berries, nuts and seeds – and for some people, even legumes. You do this by adding just 5 g of Net Carbs per day in weekly increments until weight loss ceases. So you go from 20 to 25 g per day one week, then to 30 g daily the next week and so forth. Then drop back 5 g and you've discovered the amount of carbs you can eat while still losing weight. For most people, that amount is somewhere between 40 and 60 grams daily. Continue until you are within 2.25 to 4.5 kg/5 to 10 lb of your goal weight.

Phase 3: Pre-Maintenance. With your goal in sight, you'll want to slow your weight loss to an almost imperceptible rate so that your good eating habits become ingrained. Each week, you'll now add another 10 g of daily Net Carbs to your programme – or treat yourself to an extra 20 to 30 g of nutrient-dense Net Carbs twice a week – so long as you continue to lose. If your weight loss stops, cut back 5 or 10 g until you resume gradual weight loss. This is your revised level for carb consumption, at which you will continue until you reach your target weight.

Phase 4: Lifetime Maintenance. Now that you've achieved your goal weight, you can start enjoying an even wider range of delicious foods. You still need to keep an eye on your carb intake, of course. Is that hard to do? No. Just skip the junk food and use your carb grams on nutrient-rich foods such as whole, unrefined grains and a variety of fruits and vegetables. Most people find that they can maintain their weight by consuming somewhere between 60 and 120 g of Net Carbs a day. Someone who is fit and exercises an hour or more daily may be able to go even higher. This individualized number is your Atkins Carbohydrate Equilibrium (ACE), the number of grams of Net Carbs you can eat without gaining or losing weight. This is your equilibrium zone in which you'll maintain your weight effortlessly while eating a satisfying, healthful diet.

For more on all four phases of the Atkins Nutritional Approach, read *Dr Atkins New Diet Revolution* or go to www.atkins.com.

Phase 1: Induction

To ensure success doing Atkins you must follow the first phase precisely. This helps you kick-start weight loss. Any variance or rationalizations such as 'just this one taste won't hurt' may interfere with results, which could in turn affect your commitment to stay with the programme.

What Are Net Carbs?

The only carbs that matter when you do Atkins are Net Carbs as these are the ones that have a significant effect on blood sugar. They are called Net Carbs because they represent total carb grams minus the grams of carbs that don't impact blood sugar. In the USA, Net Carbs reflect total carbs minus fibre and certain carbohydrates like polyols (sugar alcohols), including glycerine and malitol, which act as sweeteners. Because food labels in the UK distinguish the fibre content from the carb content, if there are no sugar alcohols in a product, the number of grams of total carbohydrates and of Net Carbs is the same. But if you are looking at labels on foods from countries that list fibre as a carbohydrate, make sure to subtract the grams of fibre from the carbohydrate grams to get the Net Carb count. In the case of unprocessed foods such as vegetables and berries, you may need to use a carbohydrate gram counter (such as *Dr Atkins New Carbohydrate Counter*). If the gram counter includes fibre in its totals, subtract the fibre from the total carb count.

The Right Way to Do Induction

To achieve speedy weight loss while feeling good, follow these 20 rules of Induction to the letter:

1. Do not skip meals. You can eat three normal-sized meals a day or four or five smaller meals.

2. Do not go more than six waking hours without eating.

3. Eat enough protein in the form of poultry, fish, shellfish, eggs and red meat to feel comfortably full but not stuffed.

4. Eat liberal amounts of natural fats, such as olive oil, butter, mayonnaise, avocado, and sunflower and other vegetable oils (preferably expeller-pressed or cold-pressed). You need not trim fat from meat or poultry.

5. Avoid hydrogenated fats, which contain trans fats.

6. Eat no more than 20 g a day of Net Carbs, in the form of 3 small handfuls of salad greens or 2 small handfuls of greens and 2 tablespoons of other vegetables.

7. Eat no fruit, bread, pasta, grains, starchy vegetables or legumes.

8. Eat no dairy products other than cheese, cream or butter.

9. Do not eat nuts or seeds in the first two weeks.

10. Eat only food on the Acceptable Foods list.

11. Let your appetite be your guide. Eat when you're hungry but stop as soon as you are pleasantly full.

12. Have a small low carb snack if you are hungry between meals.

13. If you're not hungry at mealtime eat a small low carb snack with your nutritional supplements.

14. Don't assume any food is low carbohydrate. Check the carb count on every packet (be sure your serving size corresponds to that listed) and/or use a carbohydrate gram counter.

15. When you eat out, watch for hidden carbs. Flour, cornflour and sugar are often in gravies, sauces and dressings.

16. Use sucralose (Splenda) or saccharin (Hermestas, Sweetex) as a sweetener. Be sure to count each packet as 1 g of Net Carbs.

17. Avoid caffeine in the form of coffee, tea and soft drinks. Excessive caffeine can cause low blood sugar, making you crave sugar.

18. Drink at least eight 225-ml/8-fl oz glasses of water each day.

19. If you are constipated, mix a tablespoon or more of psyllium husks in 225 ml/8 fl oz or more of water and drink daily. Or mix ground flaxseeds into a shake or sprinkle wheat bran over a salad or vegetables. Fibre need not be counted in your daily carb count (see page 217).

20. Take a good daily multivitamin with minerals – including potassium, magnesium and calcium – as well as an essential fatty acids supplement.

Acceptable Foods in Induction

You can eat the following foods liberally during the first phase:

All fish   **All poultry**

All shellfish   **All red meat**

All eggs

Special Considerations:

- Oysters and mussels are higher in carbs than other shellfish, so eat no more than 115 g/4 oz a day.
- Processed meats, such as ham, bacon, pepperoni, salami, hot dogs and other luncheon meats – and some fish – may be cured with sugar or contain fillers that contribute carbs.
- Avoid meat and fish products cured with nitrates, which are known carcinogens. Also be wary of products that are not exclusively meat, fish or fowl, such as imitation crabmeat, fish sticks, meatloaf and breaded foods.
- Do not consume more than 115 g/4 oz of offal a day.

Special Category Foods

Each day you can also eat the following:

- 10 to 20 olives
- Half a small avocado
- 30 ml/1 fl oz of soured cream or 90 ml/3 oz of unsweetened double cream
- 2 to 3 tablespoons of lemon juice or lime juice

Note that these foods occasionally slow down weight loss in some people, and may need to be avoided in the first two weeks. If you seem to be losing slowly, moderate your intake of these foods.

Other Acceptable Foods During Induction

CHEESE

You can consume 85 to 115 g/3 to 4 oz daily of the following full-fat, firm, soft and semi-soft aged cheeses, including:

Cheddar	Sheep and goat cheese
Cream cheese	Gouda
Mozzarella	Gruyère or Emmenthal
Roquefort and other blue cheeses	

Special Considerations:
- All cheeses contain some carbohydrates. The rule of thumb is to count 25 g/1 oz of cheese as equivalent to 1 g of Net Carbs.
- Note that cottage cheese and other fresh cheeses are not permitted during Induction. Nor are 'diet' or whey cheeses, or processed cheeses such as cheese spreads
- Soya or rice 'cheeses' are permitted but check the carb content.

SALAD VEGETABLES

You can have 2 to 3 small handfuls per day of the following raw vegetables:

Chicory	Endive
Escarole	Lamb's Lettuce
Lettuce	Radicchio
Rocket	Romaine (Cos)
Sorrel	Spinach

or 4 to 6 tablespoons of the following raw vegetables:

Alfalfa Sprouts	Celery
Chives	Cucumber
Daikon	Fennel
Mushrooms	Parsley

| Peppers | Radishes |
| Spring Onions | |

OTHER VEGETABLES

You can have 2 tablespoons per day of these cooked veggies if salad does not exceed 2 small handfuls/4 tablespoons:

Artichoke	Artichoke hearts
Asparagus	Aubergine
Bamboo shoots	Bean sprouts
Beet greens	Broccoli
Brussels Spouts	Cabbage
Cauliflower	Celeriac
Chard	Courgettes
Dandelion greens	Hearts of palm
Kale	Kohlrabi
Leeks	Mange-tout
Okra	Onion
Pak Choy	Pumpkin
Rhubarb	Runner or wax beans
Sauerkraut	Spaghetti squash
Summer Squash	Tomato
Turnips	Water Chestnuts

Special Considerations:
- If a vegetable (e.g. tomato) cooks down significantly, measure it raw so you don't underestimate its carb count.

SALAD GARNISHES

Crumbled crisp bacon	Grated cheese
Sautéed mushrooms	Soured cream
Chopped hard-boiled egg	

Note: Use spices and herbs to taste, but make sure none contain added sugar.

SALAD DRESSINGS

- Avoid prepared salad dressings with added sugar.
- Use oil and vinegar (but not balsamic vinegar, which contains sugar) or lemon juice and herbs and spices.
- Use only prepared dressings with no more than 2 g of Net Carbs per tablespoon serving.

ACCEPTABLE FATS AND OILS

Olive oil	Rapeseed oil
Walnut oil	Soya bean oil
Grapeseed oil	Sesame oil
Sunflower oil	Safflower oil

Butter (Avoid margarine made with trans fats)

ARTIFICIAL SWEETENERS

Sucralose
  (marketed as Splenda)
Saccharin
  (marketed as Hermestas and Sweetex)

Special Considerations:
- Avoid natural sweeteners ending in the suffix '-ose', such as maltose, fructose, etc. Sugar alcohols, such as maltitol, do not affect blood sugar and are acceptable.

Acceptable Beverages

Be sure to drink a minimum of eight 225-ml/8-fl oz glasses of water each day, including:

Filtered water	**Mineral water**
Spring water	**Tap water**

Additionally, you can have the following:

- Clear broth/bouillon (not all brands; read the label)
- Soda water
- Cream, double or single (limit to 2 to 3 tablespoons a day; note carb content)
- Decaffeinated coffee or tea
- Diet soda made with sucralose (Splenda); be sure to count the carbs
- Essence-flavoured water (must say 'no calories')
- Herb tea (without barley sugar or any fruit sugar added)
- Lemon juice or lime juice (note that each contains 2.8 g carbohydrate per 25 g/1 oz); limit to 2 to 3 tablespoons

---

Special Considerations:
- Grain beverages (coffee substitutes) are not allowed.
- Alcoholic beverages are not permitted during Induction.

Convenience Foods

You can also select from the variety of convenience foods, but always check labels to find the Net Carbs in any particular product. Atkins convenience food products suitable for Induction include:

Atkins Advantage™ Bars
Each 60 g bar contains 2-3 g of Net Carbs.

Atkins Advantage™ Ready-to-Drink Shakes
Each 330 ml can contains 2 g of Net Carbs.

Atkins Morning Shine™ Breakfast Bars
Each 185 g bar contains 3 g of Net Carbs.

To find a retailer of Atkins Nutritional Products in your area, go to www.atkins.com. Additional products are also available for purchase online.

What Are Net Carbs?

Not all carbohydrates labelled on food and beverage products have the same metabolic effect on our bodies. Unlike typical carbohydrates, fibre, glycerine and sugar alcohols have a have a minimal impact on blood sugar levels. That's why Net Carbs subtract these components from the total carb count. Net Carbs are the only carbs you need to count when doing Atkins. (For more information on Net Carbs in the UK see also page 20.)

When Can I Move Beyond Induction?

You should stay on Induction for a minimum of two weeks. If you have a lot of weight to lose or have difficulty losing weight, you might want to stay on it longer. That way you'll see dramatic progress before moving on to the more moderate phases of Atkins.

In order to decide if this is the right time for you to move on, ask yourself the following four questions:

1. **Am I bored with Induction?** Boredom could lead to not complying with the rules of Induction. If you are bored by the food choices in Induction, by all means move on to OWL after two weeks.

2. **How much weight do I have to lose?** If you still have a lot to lose, you can safely stay with Induction for six months or more. If your weight goals are modest, it's advisable to advance to OWL so you can cycle through all the phases of the programme.

3. **Am I metabolically resistant to weight loss?** People with high metabolic resistance lose weight relatively slowly. They can benefit from doing Induction longer because it gives them time to correct metabolic imbalances they may have developed over time. These include insulin resistance, blood sugar imbalances,

carbohydrate addictions and allergies. Once the metabolic imbalances are corrected, weight loss may speed up.

4. **Am I willing to slow down the pace of weight loss in exchange for more food choices?** If you are the type to just go for it, you may decide to stick with it until you drop some more weight. On the other hand, if you want to relax a bit about food choices, you might choose to move to the more liberal phase of OWL. Ultimately, it's a matter of whether you're willing to trade a longer time to get to your goal weight for more food choices. It's up to you.

The decision about whether to stay on Induction or move to Ongoing Weight Loss is yours alone and is another example of how much individualization is possible on Atkins.

Phase 2: Ongoing Weight Loss

When you move on to Ongoing Weight Loss (OWL), you add carbohydrate, in the form of nutrient-dense and fibre-rich foods, by increasing to 25 g of Net Carbs daily the first week, 30 g daily the next week and so on until weight loss stops. Then subtract 5 g of Net Carbs from your daily intake so that you continue sustained, moderate weight loss.

When you do Atkins, your rate of weight loss is generally proportional to the amount of carbohydrate you consume. Once you know the number of grams of Net Carbs in a certain food, you know how much you can safely eat. Fortunately, counting is easy with the help of a carbohydrate gram counter. *Dr Atkins New Carbohydrate Counter* lists Net Carbs as well as total carbs for more than 1,000 common foods.

Your daily threshold of carbohydrate consumption is called your Critical Carbohydrate Level for Losing (CCLL). Stay below this number and you will experience ongoing weight loss. Exceed it and weight loss will stall.

The Right Way to Do OWL

To be successful on the second phase of Atkins, follow these rules:

1. Protein and fat remain the mainstays of your diet.

2. Count your daily grams of Net Carbs.

3. Read food labels.

4. Use a carb gram counter.

5. Increase your daily Net Carb intake by no more than 5 g each week.

6. Increase your Net Carb intake only if you continue to lose weight.

7. If you gain weight or stop losing, drop back 5 g of Net Carbs a day until weight loss resumes.

8. Add only one new food group at a time.

9. Eat a food group no more than three times per week to start, and then eat it daily.

10. Stop eating new foods immediately if they lead to weight gain.

11. Stop new foods if physical symptoms lost during Induction return.

12. Stop new foods if they lead to increased appetite or cravings.

13. Drink eight 225-ml/8-fl oz glasses of water a day.

14. Continue to take a good multivitamin/mineral and an essential fatty acids supplement.

15. Continue doing OWL until you have 2.25 to 4.5 kg/ 5 to 10 lb left to lose.

The Power of Five

These portions contain roughly 5 g of Net Carbs. Food groups are arranged in the general order in which they should be added back during Ongoing Weight Loss.

VEGETABLES

4 tablespoons cooked spinach
3 tablespoons raw, chopped red peppers
1 medium tomato
4 tablespoons cooked broccoli florets
12 medium asparagus spears
4 tablespoons cooked cauliflower florets
2 tablespoons chopped onion
½ avocado
6 tablespoons steamed courgette slices

DAIRY

140 g/5 oz cream cheese*
140 g/5 oz mozzarella cheese
125 g/4½ oz cottage cheese*
250 g/8½ oz ricotta cheese*
170 ml/6 fl oz double cream

* Although these foods are low in carbohydrate they are not permitted during Induction. They can be eaten in moderation in later phases.

NUTS & SEEDS

Because nuts and seeds are so rich and generally low in carbs, the following servings provide no more than 3 g of Net Carbs.

25 g/1 oz of:
  Macadamias (approximately 10 to 12 nuts)
  Walnuts (approximately 14 halves)
  Almonds (approximately 14 nuts)
  Pecans (approximately 14 halves)
  Hulled sunflower seeds (3 tablespoons)
  Roasted shelled peanuts (approximately 26 nuts)
15 g/½ oz of:
  Cashews (approximately 9 nuts)

BERRIES & FRUITS

  2 tablespoons raspberries (fresh)
  2 tablespoons strawberries (fresh)
  1 tablespoon cantaloupe or honeydew melon
  1 small plum

JUICES

  60 ml/2 fl oz lemon juice
  60 ml/2 fl oz lime juice
  120 ml/4 fl oz tomato juice

Replacement Foods

Many Atkins products were designed with the OWL phase of the Atkins Nutritional Approach in mind and can now be incorporated into your eating plan along with those that are appropriate for Induction (see page 28). These items tend to be higher in protein and fibre and lower in carbohydrates than their conventional alternatives.

Atkins replacement foods suitable for OWL and beyond include:

Endulge Chocolate Candy	**Each bar contains 2–3 g of Net Carbs**
Atkins Crunchers Chips	**Each 25 g bag contains 4–5 g of Net Carbs**
Atkins Hot Cereal:	**Each packet contains 5–6 g of Net Carbs**
Atkins Pasta Cuts	**Each 55 g serving contains 6 g of Net Carbs**
Atkins Fajitas	**Each fajita contains 7–8 g of Net Carbs**
Atkins Savory Sides	**Each serving contains 4 g of Net Carbs**

Atkins Mini-Cheesecakes	**Each cake contains 3–4 g of Net Carbs**
Atkins Kitchen Fudge Brownie Mix	**Each brownie contains 4 g of Net Carbs**

To buy these products online or to find a retailer of Atkins Nutritionals products in your area, go to www.atkins.com.

Phase 3: Pre-Maintenance

Make the transition from weight loss to weight maintenance by increasing your daily intake in increments of 10 g of Net Carbs each week so long as very gradual weight loss continues.

The Right Way to Do Pre-Maintenance

To ensure success on Phase 3 of the Atkins Nutritional Approach, follow these rules:

1. Increase your daily Net Carb intake by no more than 10 g of Net Carbs each week so long as you continue to lose weight.

2. Be sure to continue eating adequate amounts of fat and protein even as the proportion of each diminishes slightly as part of your overall diet.

3. Continue to count your daily intake of grams of Net Carbs.

4. Continue to use a carb gram counter.

5. Continue to read food labels.

6. Add only one new food group at a time.

7. Eat a food group no more than three times per week to start, and then eat it daily.

8. Introduce new carbohydrate foods individually.

9. Eliminate a new food if it provokes weight gain.

10. Likewise, stop eating a new food if it prompts return of physical symptoms lost during Induction.

11. Stop eating a new food if it leads to increased appetite or cravings.

12. If you gain weight or fail to continue to lose, drop back 5 g of Net Carbs until weight loss resumes.

13. Continue to drink eight 225-ml/8-fl oz glasses of water a day.

14. Continue to take a good multivitamin/mineral and an essential fatty acids supplement.

15. Stay on Pre-Maintenance until you have maintained your goal weight for one month.

Phase 4: Lifetime Maintenance

Select from a wide variety of foods while controlling carbohydrate intake to ensure weight maintenance and a sense of well-being. Once you've reached your goal weight and are in Phase 4 of Atkins, here's how to stay there for good.

The Right Way to Do Lifetime Maintenance

1. Make weight control a constant priority.

2. Be food smart. Fresh fish, fowl, meat and nutrient-dense carbohydrates, such as vegetables, nuts, seeds and occasional fruits and starches are the foods nature intended you to eat, not the packaged refined stuff.

3. Be wary of sugar, corn syrup, honey, white flour and cornflour. Look at the labels of any packaged food you are considering and avoid any with these ingredients.

4. Try new foods to increase the variety of foods that you like and enjoy and avoid boredom. They will help prevent you from going back to eating foods that you have enjoyed in the past, but which simply aren't good for you.

5. Use low carb alternatives, as well as the recipes provided on www.atkins.com. Once you're happy with eating healthy foods, your nutritional future is almost assuredly going to be a healthy one.

6. Learn your Atkins Carbohydrate Equilibrium (ACE) and stick to it. (See page 19.)

7. Continue your programme of vitamin and mineral supplementation, including essential oils.

8. Continue to drink at least eight 225-ml/8-fl oz glasses of water a day.

9. Consume caffeine and alcohol only in moderation.

10. Never allow yourself to be more than 2.25 kg/ 5 lb away from your goal weight. Take care of weight regain promptly by dropping back one or more levels in grams of Net Carb intake until you start losing again. You may even have to return to Induction for five to seven days to stop cravings and regain control. Once you have gotten back to your goal weight, remain at your ACE.

11. Don't fall back on your former bad habits. Develop a strategy for dealing with temptation. Don't use food to alleviate stress or to cheer yourself up. Find ways other than food to 'treat' yourself.

12. Develop strategies for dealing with everyday challenges such as dining out and taking vacations. (See page 219.)

13. Make exercise a regular part of your life.

14. Get rid of your 'fat' wardrobe.

15. Weigh yourself at least once a week.

Shopping List

The best way to stick with Atkins is to have plenty of low carb foods and meal ingredients in your cupboards, refrigerator and freezer. The following items provide the basis for many a tasty meal.

FREEZER

Spinach
Chopped kale
Mange-tout or sugar snaps
Green beans
Artichoke hearts
Asparagus spears
Chopped broccoli
Unsweetened strawberries
Unsweetened blueberries
Unsweetened raspberries
Rhubarb
Frozen cooked prawns
Frozen crab meat (not artificial 'crab product')

REFRIGERATOR

Cheese (cottage cheese, ricotta, goat's cheese and mascarpone, Brie, Camembert, Gruyère, Parmesan, Gouda, cheddar, Roquefort, Gorgonzola)
Cream/butter
Eggs
Protein (poultry, fish and red meat)

Cold cuts (when possible, buy fresh from the deli counter
rather than prepackaged)
Salad vegetables
Vegetables/fruits
Tofu

FRESH HERBS

Basil
Chives
Coriander
Parsley (flat-leaf, also known as Italian, is more flavoursome
than curly parsley)
Spring onions
Ginger (a root, not a herb)

CONDIMENTS

Canned chillies (to add zip to baked dishes or mild sauces)
Tabasco sauce
Worcestershire sauce
Reduced-sodium soy sauce
Capers
Mustard (country-style or Dijon)
Sugar-free ketchup
Sugar-free barbecue sauce
White horseradish
Pesto
Canned or jarred anchovies
Vinegars (white wine, red wine, tarragon and rice wine)
Safflower or peanut oil
Olive oil
Mayonnaise (regular, full fat)

SPICES

Cajun spice blend
Chilli flakes
Chilli powder
Chinese five-spice powder (this mix of cinnamon, star anise, cloves, fennel seeds and pepper gives Chinese food its distinctive flavour)
Cinnamon
Cumin
Curry powder
Garlic powder
Marjoram (a more delicate version of oregano)
Nutmeg
Oregano
Rosemary
Sage
Tarragon
Thyme

MEAL BUILDERS

Canned reduced-sodium beef, chicken and vegetable broths
Boxed tomato sauce and chopped tomatoes
Tomato purée
Sun-dried tomatoes in oil
Dried porcini mushrooms
Tinned pumpkin
Wild rice
Cornmeal
Marinated artichoke hearts
Roasted red peppers

CANNED PROTEIN

Tuna packed in oil or water
Salmon
Sardines
Canned black soya beans
Poached white-meat chicken

NUTS, SEEDS AND NUT BUTTERS

Macadamia nuts
Almonds
Walnuts
Hazelnuts
Pecans
Sunflower seeds
Pumpkin seeds
Macadamia or almond butter (unsweetened)
Peanut butter (unsweetened)

BAKING BASICS AND SWEET ITEMS

Cocoa powder and unsweetened chocolate
Sugar substitute in granular form
Low carbohydrate sugar-free pancake syrup
Low carbohydrate bake mix
Extracts (vanilla, chocolate, banana, hazelnut, almond and coconut)
Flavoured citrus oils
Sugar-free jams

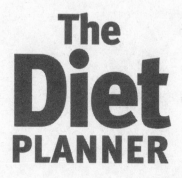

The Diet PLANNER

A 120-Day Record

Week
1

Day 1

NET CARB LEVEL:

Phase:

NET CARB
COUNT:

Breakfast:

Lunch:

Dinner:

Snacks:

Beverages:

TOTAL DAILY NET CARBS:

Supplements taken:

Water Intake:

Exercise:

Day 2

NET CARB LEVEL:

Phase:

**NET CARB
COUNT:**

Breakfast:

Lunch:

Dinner:

Snacks:

Beverages:

TOTAL DAILY NET CARBS:

Supplements taken:

Water Intake:

Exercise:

Day 3

NET CARB LEVEL: ◯

Phase:

NET CARB COUNT:

Breakfast:

Lunch:

Dinner:

Snacks:

Beverages:

TOTAL DAILY NET CARBS: ◯

Supplements taken:

Water Intake:

Exercise:

Day 4

NET CARB LEVEL:

Phase:

NET CARB COUNT:

Breakfast:

Lunch:

Dinner:

Snacks:

Beverages:

TOTAL DAILY NET CARBS:

Supplements taken:

Water Intake:

Exercise:

Day 5

NET CARB LEVEL:

Phase:

NET CARB COUNT:

Breakfast:

Lunch:

Dinner:

Snacks:

Beverages:

TOTAL DAILY NET CARBS:

Supplements taken:

Water Intake:

Exercise:

Day 6

NET CARB LEVEL:

Phase:

NET CARB
COUNT:

Breakfast:

Lunch:

Dinner:

Snacks:

Beverages:

TOTAL DAILY NET CARBS:

Supplements taken:

Water Intake:

Exercise:

Day 7

NET CARB LEVEL:

Phase:

NET CARB
COUNT:

Breakfast:

Lunch:

Dinner:

Snacks:

Beverages:

TOTAL DAILY NET CARBS:

Supplements taken:

Water Intake:

Exercise:

Week 1

TAKING STOCK

Weight

Measurements

BUST/CHEST:

WAIST:

HIPS:

UPPER ARMS:

THIGHS:

Rate the Following

Sticking to the programme
- ❏ excellent
- ❏ good
- ❏ need help

Exercise
- ❏ daily
- ❏ 1–3x/week
- ❏ nonexistent

Taking supplements
- ❏ always
- ❏ sometimes
- ❏ never

Mood
- ❏ positive
- ❏ neutral
- ❏ negative

Energy
- ❏ high
- ❏ medium
- ❏ low

Did you have cravings this week? Did you try to resist them? Were you successful?

What other challenges did you face this week?

Were you able to overcome them? If so, how? If not, what might help you do so?

Did you face any stressful situations? How did they affect your adherence to the programme?

What new foods/recipes did you add this week?

What is working for you? What changes do you need to make?

Week

2

Day 8

NET CARB LEVEL:

Phase:

NET CARB COUNT:

Breakfast:

Lunch:

Dinner:

Snacks:

Beverages:

TOTAL DAILY NET CARBS:

Supplements taken:

Water Intake:

Exercise:

Day 9

NET CARB LEVEL: ⬭

Phase:

NET CARB
COUNT:

Breakfast:

Lunch:

Dinner:

Snacks:

Beverages:

TOTAL DAILY NET CARBS: ⬭

Supplements taken:

Water Intake:

Exercise:

Day 10

NET CARB LEVEL: ⬭

Phase:

NET CARB COUNT:

Breakfast:

Lunch:

Dinner:

Snacks:

Beverages:

TOTAL DAILY NET CARBS: ⬭

Supplements taken:

Water Intake:

Exercise:

Day 11

NET CARB LEVEL:

Phase:

NET CARB COUNT:

Breakfast:

Lunch:

Dinner:

Snacks:

Beverages:

TOTAL DAILY NET CARBS:

Supplements taken:

Water Intake:

Exercise:

Day 12

NET CARB LEVEL: ⬭

Phase:

NET CARB COUNT:

Breakfast:

Lunch:

Dinner:

Snacks:

Beverages:

TOTAL DAILY NET CARBS: ⬭

Supplements taken:

Water Intake:

Exercise:

Day 13

NET CARB LEVEL: ◯

Phase:

NET CARB COUNT:

Breakfast:

Lunch:

Dinner:

Snacks:

Beverages:

TOTAL DAILY NET CARBS: ◯

Supplements taken:

Water Intake:

Exercise:

Day 14

NET CARB LEVEL:

Phase:

NET CARB
COUNT:

Breakfast:

Lunch:

Dinner:

Snacks:

Beverages:

TOTAL DAILY NET CARBS:

Supplements taken:

Water Intake:

Exercise:

Week 2

TAKING STOCK

Weight

Measurements

BUST/CHEST:

WAIST:

HIPS:

UPPER ARMS:

THIGHS:

Rate the Following

Sticking to the programme
- ❏ excellent
- ❏ good
- ❏ need help

Exercise
- ❏ daily
- ❏ 1–3x/week
- ❏ nonexistent

Taking supplements
- ❏ always
- ❏ sometimes
- ❏ never

Mood
- ❏ positive
- ❏ neutral
- ❏ negative

Energy
- ❏ high
- ❏ medium
- ❏ low

Did you have cravings this week? Did you try to resist them? Were you successful?

What other challenges did you face this week?

Were you able to overcome them? If so, how? If not, what might help you do so?

Did you face any stressful situations? How did they affect your adherence to the programme?

What new foods/recipes did you add this week?

What is working for you? What changes do you need to make?

Week

3

Day 15

Today's date is:

NET CARB LEVEL: ⬭

Phase:

NET CARB COUNT:

Breakfast:

Lunch:

Dinner:

Snacks:

Beverages:

TOTAL DAILY NET CARBS: ⬭

Supplements taken:

Water Intake:

Exercise:

Day 16

Today's date is:

NET CARB LEVEL:

Phase:

NET CARB
COUNT:

Breakfast:

Lunch:

Dinner:

Snacks:

Beverages:

TOTAL DAILY NET CARBS:

Supplements taken:

Water Intake:

Exercise:

Day 17

NET CARB LEVEL: ⬭

Phase:

NET CARB COUNT:

Breakfast:

Lunch:

Dinner:

Snacks:

Beverages:

TOTAL DAILY NET CARBS: ⬭

Supplements taken:

Water Intake:

Exercise:

Day 18

NET CARB LEVEL:

Phase:

NET CARB COUNT:

Breakfast:

Lunch:

Dinner:

Snacks:

Beverages:

TOTAL DAILY NET CARBS:

Supplements taken:

Water Intake:

Exercise:

Day 19

Today's date is:

NET CARB LEVEL:

Phase:

NET CARB COUNT:

Breakfast:

Lunch:

Dinner:

Snacks:

Beverages:

TOTAL DAILY NET CARBS:

Supplements taken:

Water Intake:

Exercise:

Day 20

NET CARB LEVEL: ⬭

Phase:

NET CARB
COUNT:

Breakfast:

Lunch:

Dinner:

Snacks:

Beverages:

TOTAL DAILY NET CARBS: ⬭

Supplements taken:

Water Intake:

Exercise:

Day 21

NET CARB LEVEL: ⬭

Phase:

NET CARB COUNT:

Breakfast:

Lunch:

Dinner:

Snacks:

Beverages:

TOTAL DAILY NET CARBS: ⬭

Supplements taken:

Water Intake:

Exercise:

Week 3

TAKING STOCK

Weight

Measurements

BUST/CHEST:

WAIST:

HIPS:

UPPER ARMS: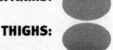

THIGHS:

Rate the Following

Sticking to the programme
- ❏ excellent
- ❏ good
- ❏ need help

Exercise
- ❏ daily
- ❏ 1–3x/week
- ❏ nonexistent

Taking supplements
- ❏ always
- ❏ sometimes
- ❏ never

Mood
- ❏ positive
- ❏ neutral
- ❏ negative

Energy
- ❏ high
- ❏ medium
- ❏ low

Did you have cravings this week? Did you try to resist them? Were you successful?

What other challenges did you face this week?

Were you able to overcome them? If so, how? If not, what might help you do so?

Did you face any stressful situations? How did they affect your adherence to the programme?

What new foods/recipes did you add this week?

What is working for you? What changes do you need to make?

Week
4

Day 22

NET CARB LEVEL:

Phase:

NET CARB COUNT:

Breakfast:

Lunch:

Dinner:

Snacks:

Beverages:

TOTAL DAILY NET CARBS:

Supplements taken:

Water Intake:

Exercise:

Day 23

NET CARB LEVEL:

Phase:

NET CARB COUNT:

Breakfast:

Lunch:

Dinner:

Snacks:

Beverages:

TOTAL DAILY NET CARBS:

Supplements taken:

Water Intake:

Exercise:

Day 24

NET CARB LEVEL:

Phase:

NET CARB COUNT:

Breakfast:

Lunch:

Dinner:

Snacks:

Beverages:

TOTAL DAILY NET CARBS:

Supplements taken:

Water Intake:

Exercise:

Day 25

NET CARB LEVEL:

Phase:

NET CARB COUNT:

Breakfast:

Lunch:

Dinner:

Snacks:

Beverages:

TOTAL DAILY NET CARBS:

Supplements taken:

Water Intake:

Exercise:

Day 26

NET CARB LEVEL: ⬭

Phase:

NET CARB COUNT:

Breakfast:

Lunch:

Dinner:

Snacks:

Beverages:

TOTAL DAILY NET CARBS: ⬭

Supplements taken:

Water Intake:

Exercise:

Day 27

NET CARB LEVEL:

Phase:

NET CARB COUNT:

Breakfast:

Lunch:

Dinner:

Snacks:

Beverages:

TOTAL DAILY NET CARBS:

Supplements taken:

Water Intake:

Exercise:

Day 28

NET CARB LEVEL:

Phase:

NET CARB COUNT:

Breakfast:

Lunch:

Dinner:

Snacks:

Beverages:

TOTAL DAILY NET CARBS:

Supplements taken:

Water Intake:

Exercise:

Week 4

TAKING STOCK

Weight

Measurements

BUST/CHEST: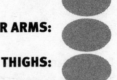

WAIST:

HIPS:

UPPER ARMS:

THIGHS:

Rate the Following

Sticking to the programme
- ❏ excellent
- ❏ good
- ❏ need help

Exercise
- ❏ daily
- ❏ 1–3x/week
- ❏ nonexistent

Taking supplements
- ❏ always
- ❏ sometimes
- ❏ never

Mood
- ❏ positive
- ❏ neutral
- ❏ negative

Energy
- ❏ high
- ❏ medium
- ❏ low

Did you have cravings this week? Did you try to resist them? Were you successful?

What other challenges did you face this week?

Were you able to overcome them? If so, how? If not, what might help you do so?

Did you face any stressful situations? How did they affect your adherence to the programme?

What new foods/recipes did you add this week?

What is working for you? What changes do you need to make?

Week

5

Day 29

NET CARB LEVEL:

Phase:

NET CARB
COUNT:

Breakfast:

Lunch:

Dinner:

Snacks:

Beverages:

TOTAL DAILY NET CARBS:

Supplements taken:

Water Intake:

Exercise:

Day 30

NET CARB LEVEL:

Phase:

NET CARB COUNT:

Breakfast:

Lunch:

Dinner:

Snacks:

Beverages:

TOTAL DAILY NET CARBS:

Supplements taken:

Water Intake:

Exercise:

Day 31

NET CARB LEVEL:

Phase:

NET CARB COUNT:

Breakfast:

Lunch:

Dinner:

Snacks:

Beverages:

TOTAL DAILY NET CARBS:

Supplements taken:

Water Intake:

Exercise:

Day 32

Today's date is:

NET CARB LEVEL: ◯

Phase:

NET CARB
COUNT:

Breakfast: ⬤

Lunch: ⬤

Dinner: ⬤

Snacks: ⬤

Beverages: ⬤

TOTAL DAILY NET CARBS: ◯

Supplements taken:

Water Intake:

Exercise:

Day 33

NET CARB LEVEL:

Phase:

NET CARB COUNT:

Breakfast:

Lunch:

Dinner:

Snacks:

Beverages:

TOTAL DAILY NET CARBS:

Supplements taken:

Water Intake:

Exercise:

Day 34

NET CARB LEVEL:

Phase:

NET CARB COUNT:

Breakfast:

Lunch:

Dinner:

Snacks:

Beverages:

TOTAL DAILY NET CARBS:

Supplements taken:

Water Intake:

Exercise:

Day 35

NET CARB LEVEL: $\bigcirc$

Phase:

NET CARB COUNT:

Breakfast:

Lunch:

Dinner:

Snacks:

Beverages:

TOTAL DAILY NET CARBS: $\bigcirc$

Supplements taken:

Water Intake:

Exercise:

Week 5

TAKING STOCK

Weight

Measurements

BUST/CHEST: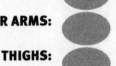

WAIST:

HIPS:

UPPER ARMS:

THIGHS:

Rate the Following

Sticking to the programme
- ❏ excellent
- ❏ good
- ❏ need help

Exercise
- ❏ daily
- ❏ 1–3x/week
- ❏ nonexistent

Taking supplements
- ❏ always
- ❏ sometimes
- ❏ never

Mood
- ❏ positive
- ❏ neutral
- ❏ negative

Energy
- ❏ high
- ❏ medium
- ❏ low

Did you have cravings this week? Did you try to resist them? Were you successful?

What other challenges did you face this week?

Were you able to overcome them? If so, how? If not, what might help you do so?

Did you face any stressful situations? How did they affect your adherence to the programme?

What new foods/recipes did you add this week?

What is working for you? What changes do you need to make?

Week 6

Day 36

NET CARB LEVEL:

Phase:

**NET CARB
COUNT:**

Breakfast:

Lunch:

Dinner:

Snacks:

Beverages:

TOTAL DAILY NET CARBS:

Supplements taken:

Water Intake:

Exercise:

Day 37

NET CARB LEVEL:

Phase:

NET CARB COUNT:

Breakfast:

Lunch:

Dinner:

Snacks:

Beverages:

TOTAL DAILY NET CARBS:

Supplements taken:

Water Intake:

Exercise:

Day 38

NET CARB LEVEL: ⬭

Phase:

NET CARB COUNT:

Breakfast:

Lunch:

Dinner:

Snacks:

Beverages:

TOTAL DAILY NET CARBS: ⬭

Supplements taken:

Water Intake:

Exercise:

Day 39

Today's date is:

NET CARB LEVEL:

Phase:

NET CARB COUNT:

Breakfast:

Lunch:

Dinner:

Snacks:

Beverages:

TOTAL DAILY NET CARBS:

Supplements taken:

Water Intake:

Exercise:

Day 40

NET CARB LEVEL: ⬭

Phase:

NET CARB COUNT:

Breakfast:

Lunch:

Dinner:

Snacks:

Beverages:

TOTAL DAILY NET CARBS: ⬭

Supplements taken:

Water Intake:

Exercise:

Day 41

Today's date is:

NET CARB LEVEL: ⬭

Phase:

NET CARB COUNT:

Breakfast:

Lunch:

Dinner:

Snacks:

Beverages:

TOTAL DAILY NET CARBS: ⬭

Supplements taken:

Water Intake:

Exercise:

Day 42

Today's date is:

NET CARB LEVEL:

Phase:

NET CARB COUNT:

Breakfast:

Lunch:

Dinner:

Snacks:

Beverages:

TOTAL DAILY NET CARBS:

Supplements taken:

Water Intake:

Exercise:

Week 6

TAKING STOCK

Weight

Measurements

BUST/CHEST:

WAIST:

HIPS:

UPPER ARMS:

THIGHS:

Rate the Following

Sticking to the programme
- ❑ excellent
- ❑ good
- ❑ need help

Exercise
- ❑ daily
- ❑ 1–3x/week
- ❑ nonexistent

Taking supplements
- ❑ always
- ❑ sometimes
- ❑ never

Mood
- ❑ positive
- ❑ neutral
- ❑ negative

Energy
- ❑ high
- ❑ medium
- ❑ low

Did you have cravings this week? Did you try to resist them? Were you successful?

What other challenges did you face this week?

Were you able to overcome them? If so, how? If not, what might help you do so?

Did you face any stressful situations? How did they affect your adherence to the programme?

What new foods/recipes did you add this week?

What is working for you? What changes do you need to make?

Week
7

Day 43

NET CARB LEVEL:

Phase:

NET CARB COUNT:

Breakfast:

Lunch:

Dinner:

Snacks:

Beverages:

TOTAL DAILY NET CARBS:

Supplements taken:

Water Intake:

Exercise:

Day 44

NET CARB LEVEL:

Phase:

NET CARB COUNT:

Breakfast:

Lunch:

Dinner:

Snacks:

Beverages:

TOTAL DAILY NET CARBS:

Supplements taken:

Water Intake:

Exercise:

Day 45

Today's date is:

NET CARB LEVEL: ◯

Phase:

NET CARB COUNT:

Breakfast:

Lunch:

Dinner:

Snacks:

Beverages:

TOTAL DAILY NET CARBS: ◯

Supplements taken:

Water Intake:

Exercise:

Day 46

NET CARB LEVEL: ( )

Phase:

NET CARB COUNT:

Breakfast:

Lunch:

Dinner:

Snacks:

Beverages:

TOTAL DAILY NET CARBS: ( )

Supplements taken:

Water Intake:

Exercise:

Day 47

NET CARB LEVEL: ⬭

Phase:

NET CARB COUNT:

Breakfast:

Lunch:

Dinner:

Snacks:

Beverages:

TOTAL DAILY NET CARBS: ⬭

Supplements taken:

Water Intake:

Exercise:

Day 48

NET CARB LEVEL:

Phase:

NET CARB COUNT:

Breakfast:

Lunch:

Dinner:

Snacks:

Beverages:

TOTAL DAILY NET CARBS:

Supplements taken:

Water Intake:

Exercise:

Day 49

Today's date is:

NET CARB LEVEL:

Phase:

NET CARB
COUNT:

Breakfast:

Lunch:

Dinner:

Snacks:

Beverages:

TOTAL DAILY NET CARBS:

Supplements taken:

Water Intake:

Exercise:

Week 7

TAKING STOCK

Weight

Measurements

BUST/CHEST: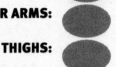

WAIST:

HIPS:

UPPER ARMS:

THIGHS:

Rate the Following

Sticking to the programme
- ❑ excellent
- ❑ good
- ❑ need help

Exercise
- ❑ daily
- ❑ 1–3x/week
- ❑ nonexistent

Taking supplements
- ❑ always
- ❑ sometimes
- ❑ never

Mood
- ❑ positive
- ❑ neutral
- ❑ negative

Energy
- ❑ high
- ❑ medium
- ❑ low

Did you have cravings this week? Did you try to resist them? Were you successful?

What other challenges did you face this week?

Were you able to overcome them? If so, how? If not, what might help you do so?

Did you face any stressful situations? How did they affect your adherence to the programme?

What new foods/recipes did you add this week?

What is working for you? What changes do you need to make?

Week 8

Day 50

NET CARB LEVEL: ⬭

Phase:

NET CARB COUNT:

Breakfast:

Lunch:

Dinner:

Snacks:

Beverages:

TOTAL DAILY NET CARBS: ⬭

Supplements taken:

Water Intake:

Exercise:

Day 51

NET CARB LEVEL:

Phase:

NET CARB COUNT:

Breakfast:

Lunch:

Dinner:

Snacks:

Beverages:

TOTAL DAILY NET CARBS:

Supplements taken:

Water Intake:

Exercise:

Day 52

Today's date is:

NET CARB LEVEL: ⬭

Phase:

NET CARB COUNT:

Breakfast:

Lunch:

Dinner:

Snacks:

Beverages:

TOTAL DAILY NET CARBS: ⬭

Supplements taken:

Water Intake:

Exercise:

Day 53

Today's date is:

NET CARB LEVEL: ⬭

Phase:

NET CARB COUNT:

Breakfast:

Lunch:

Dinner:

Snacks:

Beverages:

TOTAL DAILY NET CARBS: ⬭

Supplements taken:

Water Intake:

Exercise:

Day 54

Today's date is:

NET CARB LEVEL: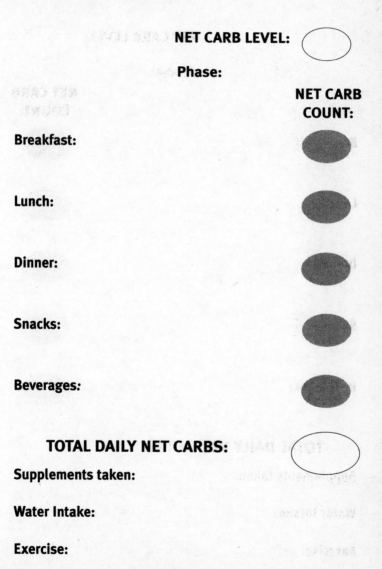

Phase:

NET CARB COUNT:

Breakfast:

Lunch:

Dinner:

Snacks:

Beverages:

TOTAL DAILY NET CARBS:

Supplements taken:

Water Intake:

Exercise:

Day 55

Today's date is:

NET CARB LEVEL:

Phase:

NET CARB COUNT:

Breakfast:

Lunch:

Dinner:

Snacks:

Beverages:

TOTAL DAILY NET CARBS:

Supplements taken:

Water Intake:

Exercise:

Day 56

NET CARB LEVEL:

Phase:

NET CARB COUNT:

Breakfast:

Lunch:

Dinner:

Snacks:

Beverages:

TOTAL DAILY NET CARBS:

Supplements taken:

Water Intake:

Exercise:

Week 8

Today's date is:

TAKING STOCK

Weight

Measurements

BUST/CHEST:

WAIST:

HIPS:

UPPER ARMS: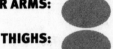

THIGHS:

Rate the Following

Sticking to the programme
- ❏ excellent
- ❏ good
- ❏ need help

Exercise
- ❏ daily
- ❏ 1–3x/week
- ❏ nonexistent

Taking supplements
- ❏ always
- ❏ sometimes
- ❏ never

Mood
- ❏ positive
- ❏ neutral
- ❏ negative

Energy
- ❏ high
- ❏ medium
- ❏ low

Did you have cravings this week? Did you try to resist them? Were you successful?

What other challenges did you face this week?

Were you able to overcome them? If so, how? If not, what might help you do so?

Did you face any stressful situations? How did they affect your adherence to the programme?

What new foods/recipes did you add this week?

What is working for you? What changes do you need to make?

Week

9

Day 57

Today's date is:

NET CARB LEVEL:

Phase:

NET CARB
COUNT:

Breakfast:

Lunch:

Dinner:

Snacks:

Beverages:

TOTAL DAILY NET CARBS:

Supplements taken:

Water Intake:

Exercise:

Day 58

NET CARB LEVEL:

Phase:

NET CARB COUNT:

Breakfast:

Lunch:

Dinner:

Snacks:

Beverages:

TOTAL DAILY NET CARBS:

Supplements taken:

Water Intake:

Exercise:

Day 59

Today's date is:

NET CARB LEVEL:

Phase:

NET CARB COUNT:

Breakfast:

Lunch:

Dinner:

Snacks:

Beverages:

TOTAL DAILY NET CARBS:

Supplements taken:

Water Intake:

Exercise:

Day 60

NET CARB LEVEL: ( )

Phase:

NET CARB COUNT:

Breakfast:

Lunch:

Dinner:

Snacks:

Beverages:

TOTAL DAILY NET CARBS: ( )

Supplements taken:

Water Intake:

Exercise:

Day 61

NET CARB LEVEL: ⬭

Phase:

NET CARB COUNT:

Breakfast:

Lunch:

Dinner:

Snacks:

Beverages:

TOTAL DAILY NET CARBS: ⬭

Supplements taken:

Water Intake:

Exercise:

Day 62

NET CARB LEVEL:

Phase:

NET CARB COUNT:

Breakfast:

Lunch:

Dinner:

Snacks:

Beverages:

TOTAL DAILY NET CARBS:

Supplements taken:

Water Intake:

Exercise:

Day 63

NET CARB LEVEL: ⬭

Phase:

NET CARB COUNT:

Breakfast: ⬬

Lunch: ⬬

Dinner: ⬬

Snacks: ⬬

Beverages: ⬬

TOTAL DAILY NET CARBS: ⬭

Supplements taken:

Water Intake:

Exercise:

Week 9

TAKING STOCK

Weight

Measurements

BUST/CHEST:

WAIST:

HIPS:

UPPER ARMS:

THIGHS:

Rate the Following

Sticking to the programme
- ❏ excellent
- ❏ good
- ❏ need help

Exercise
- ❏ daily
- ❏ 1–3x/week
- ❏ nonexistent

Taking supplements
- ❏ always
- ❏ sometimes
- ❏ never

Mood
- ❏ positive
- ❏ neutral
- ❏ negative

Energy
- ❏ high
- ❏ medium
- ❏ low

Did you have cravings this week? Did you try to resist them? Were you successful?

What other challenges did you face this week?

Were you able to overcome them? If so, how? If not, what might help you do so?

Did you face any stressful situations? How did they affect your adherence to the programme?

What new foods/recipes did you add this week?

What is working for you? What changes do you need to make?

Week

10

Day 64

NET CARB LEVEL:

Phase:

NET CARB COUNT:

Breakfast:

Lunch:

Dinner:

Snacks:

Beverages:

TOTAL DAILY NET CARBS:

Supplements taken:

Water Intake:

Exercise:

Day 65

NET CARB LEVEL:

Phase:

NET CARB COUNT:

Breakfast:

Lunch:

Dinner:

Snacks:

Beverages:

TOTAL DAILY NET CARBS:

Supplements taken:

Water Intake:

Exercise:

Day 66

NET CARB LEVEL:

Phase:

NET CARB COUNT:

Breakfast:

Lunch:

Dinner:

Snacks:

Beverages:

TOTAL DAILY NET CARBS:

Supplements taken:

Water Intake:

Exercise:

Day 67

Today's date is:

NET CARB LEVEL:

Phase:

NET CARB COUNT:

Breakfast:

Lunch:

Dinner:

Snacks:

Beverages:

TOTAL DAILY NET CARBS:

Supplements taken:

Water Intake:

Exercise:

Day 68

NET CARB LEVEL:

Phase:

NET CARB COUNT:

Breakfast:

Lunch:

Dinner:

Snacks:

Beverages:

TOTAL DAILY NET CARBS:

Supplements taken:

Water Intake:

Exercise:

Day 69

NET CARB LEVEL:

Phase:

NET CARB COUNT:

Breakfast:

Lunch:

Dinner:

Snacks:

Beverages:

TOTAL DAILY NET CARBS:

Supplements taken:

Water Intake:

Exercise:

Day 70

NET CARB LEVEL:

Phase:

NET CARB COUNT:

Breakfast:

Lunch:

Dinner:

Snacks:

Beverages:

TOTAL DAILY NET CARBS:

Supplements taken:

Water Intake:

Exercise:

Week 10

TAKING STOCK

Weight

Measurements

BUST/CHEST:

WAIST:

HIPS:

UPPER ARMS:

THIGHS:

Rate the Following

Sticking to the programme
❑ excellent
❑ good
❑ need help

Exercise
❑ daily
❑ 1–3x/week
❑ nonexistent

Taking supplements
❑ always
❑ sometimes
❑ never

Mood
❑ positive
❑ neutral
❑ negative

Energy
❑ high
❑ medium
❑ low

Did you have cravings this week? Did you try to resist them? Were you successful?

What other challenges did you face this week?

Were you able to overcome them? If so, how? If not, what might help you do so?

Did you face any stressful situations? How did they affect your adherence to the programme?

What new foods/recipes did you add this week?

What is working for you? What changes do you need to make?

Week

11

Day 71

NET CARB LEVEL:

Phase:

NET CARB COUNT:

Breakfast:

Lunch:

Dinner:

Snacks:

Beverages:

TOTAL DAILY NET CARBS:

Supplements taken:

Water Intake:

Exercise:

Day 72

NET CARB LEVEL:

Phase:

NET CARB COUNT:

Breakfast:

Lunch:

Dinner:

Snacks:

Beverages:

TOTAL DAILY NET CARBS:

Supplements taken:

Water Intake:

Exercise:

Day 73

NET CARB LEVEL: ⬭

Phase:

**NET CARB
COUNT:**

Breakfast:

Lunch:

Dinner:

Snacks:

Beverages:

TOTAL DAILY NET CARBS: ⬭

Supplements taken:

Water Intake:

Exercise:

Day 74

NET CARB LEVEL:

Phase:

NET CARB COUNT:

Breakfast:

Lunch:

Dinner:

Snacks:

Beverages:

TOTAL DAILY NET CARBS:

Supplements taken:

Water Intake:

Exercise:

Day 75

NET CARB LEVEL:

Phase:

NET CARB COUNT:

Breakfast:

Lunch:

Dinner:

Snacks:

Beverages:

TOTAL DAILY NET CARBS:

Supplements taken:

Water Intake:

Exercise:

Day 76

Today's date is:

NET CARB LEVEL:

Phase:

NET CARB COUNT:

Breakfast:

Lunch:

Dinner:

Snacks:

Beverages:

TOTAL DAILY NET CARBS:

Supplements taken:

Water Intake:

Exercise:

Day 77

NET CARB LEVEL:

Phase:

NET CARB COUNT:

Breakfast:

Lunch:

Dinner:

Snacks:

Beverages:

TOTAL DAILY NET CARBS:

Supplements taken:

Water Intake:

Exercise:

Week 11

TAKING STOCK

Weight

Measurements

BUST/CHEST:

WAIST:

HIPS:

UPPER ARMS: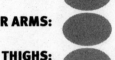

THIGHS:

Rate the Following

Sticking to the programme
- ❏ excellent
- ❏ good
- ❏ need help

Exercise
- ❏ daily
- ❏ 1–3x/week
- ❏ nonexistent

Taking supplements
- ❏ always
- ❏ sometimes
- ❏ never

Mood
- ❏ positive
- ❏ neutral
- ❏ negative

Energy
- ❏ high
- ❏ medium
- ❏ low

Did you have cravings this week? Did you try to resist them? Were you successful?

What other challenges did you face this week?

Were you able to overcome them? If so, how? If not, what might help you do so?

Did you face any stressful situations? How did they affect your adherence to the programme?

What new foods/recipes did you add this week?

What is working for you? What changes do you need to make?

Week

12

Day 78

NET CARB LEVEL:

Phase:

NET CARB COUNT:

Breakfast:

Lunch:

Dinner:

Snacks:

Beverages:

TOTAL DAILY NET CARBS:

Supplements taken:

Water Intake:

Exercise:

Day 79

Today's date is:

NET CARB LEVEL:

Phase:

NET CARB COUNT:

Breakfast:

Lunch:

Dinner:

Snacks:

Beverages:

TOTAL DAILY NET CARBS:

Supplements taken:

Water Intake:

Exercise:

Day 80

NET CARB LEVEL: ( )

Phase:

NET CARB COUNT:

Breakfast:

Lunch:

Dinner:

Snacks:

Beverages:

TOTAL DAILY NET CARBS: ( )

Supplements taken:

Water Intake:

Exercise:

Day 81

NET CARB LEVEL:

Phase:

NET CARB
COUNT:

Breakfast:

Lunch:

Dinner:

Snacks:

Beverages:

TOTAL DAILY NET CARBS:

Supplements taken:

Water Intake:

Exercise:

Day 82

NET CARB LEVEL:

Phase:

NET CARB COUNT:

Breakfast:

Lunch:

Dinner:

Snacks:

Beverages:

TOTAL DAILY NET CARBS:

Supplements taken:

Water Intake:

Exercise:

Day 83

NET CARB LEVEL:

Phase:

NET CARB COUNT:

Breakfast:

Lunch:

Dinner:

Snacks:

Beverages:

TOTAL DAILY NET CARBS:

Supplements taken:

Water Intake:

Exercise:

Day 84

NET CARB LEVEL:

Phase:

NET CARB
COUNT:

Breakfast:

Lunch:

Dinner:

Snacks:

Beverages:

TOTAL DAILY NET CARBS:

Supplements taken:

Water Intake:

Exercise:

Week 12

TAKING STOCK

Weight

Measurements

BUST/CHEST:

WAIST:

HIPS:

UPPER ARMS:

THIGHS:

Rate the Following

Sticking to the programme
- ❏ excellent
- ❏ good
- ❏ need help

Exercise
- ❏ daily
- ❏ 1–3x/week
- ❏ nonexistent

Taking supplements
- ❏ always
- ❏ sometimes
- ❏ never

Mood
- ❏ positive
- ❏ neutral
- ❏ negative

Energy
- ❏ high
- ❏ medium
- ❏ low

Did you have cravings this week? Did you try to resist them? Were you successful?

What other challenges did you face this week?

Were you able to overcome them? If so, how? If not, what might help you do so?

Did you face any stressful situations? How did they affect your adherence to the programme?

What new foods/recipes did you add this week?

What is working for you? What changes do you need to make?

Week

13

Day 85

NET CARB LEVEL:

Phase:

NET CARB
COUNT:

Breakfast:

Lunch:

Dinner:

Snacks:

Beverages:

TOTAL DAILY NET CARBS:

Supplements taken:

Water Intake:

Exercise:

Day 86

NET CARB LEVEL:

Phase:

NET CARB COUNT:

Breakfast:

Lunch:

Dinner:

Snacks:

Beverages:

TOTAL DAILY NET CARBS:

Supplements taken:

Water Intake:

Exercise:

Day 87

NET CARB LEVEL: ◯

Phase:

NET CARB COUNT:

Breakfast: ⬤

Lunch: ⬤

Dinner: ⬤

Snacks: ⬤

Beverages: ⬤

TOTAL DAILY NET CARBS: ◯

Supplements taken:

Water Intake:

Exercise:

Day 88

NET CARB LEVEL:

Phase:

NET CARB COUNT:

Breakfast:

Lunch:

Dinner:

Snacks:

Beverages:

TOTAL DAILY NET CARBS:

Supplements taken:

Water Intake:

Exercise:

Day 89

Today's date is:

NET CARB LEVEL:

Phase:

NET CARB
COUNT:

Breakfast:

Lunch:

Dinner:

Snacks:

Beverages:

TOTAL DAILY NET CARBS:

Supplements taken:

Water Intake:

Exercise:

Day 90

NET CARB LEVEL:

Phase:

NET CARB COUNT:

Breakfast:

Lunch:

Dinner:

Snacks:

Beverages:

TOTAL DAILY NET CARBS:

Supplements taken:

Water Intake:

Exercise:

Day 91

NET CARB LEVEL:

Phase:

NET CARB COUNT:

Breakfast:

Lunch:

Dinner:

Snacks:

Beverages:

TOTAL DAILY NET CARBS:

Supplements taken:

Water Intake:

Exercise:

Week 13

TAKING STOCK

Weight

Measurements

BUST/CHEST:

WAIST:

HIPS:

UPPER ARMS: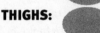

THIGHS:

Rate the Following

Sticking to the programme
- ❏ excellent
- ❏ good
- ❏ need help

Exercise
- ❏ daily
- ❏ 1–3x/week
- ❏ nonexistent

Taking supplements
- ❏ always
- ❏ sometimes
- ❏ never

Mood
- ❏ positive
- ❏ neutral
- ❏ negative

Energy
- ❏ high
- ❏ medium
- ❏ low

Did you have cravings this week? Did you try to resist them? Were you successful?

What other challenges did you face this week?

Were you able to overcome them? If so, how? If not, what might help you do so?

Did you face any stressful situations? How did they affect your adherence to the programme?

What new foods/recipes did you add this week?

What is working for you? What changes do you need to make?

Week

14

Day 92

NET CARB LEVEL: ◯

Phase:

NET CARB COUNT:

Breakfast:

Lunch:

Dinner:

Snacks:

Beverages:

TOTAL DAILY NET CARBS: ◯

Supplements taken:

Water Intake:

Exercise:

Day 93

NET CARB LEVEL:

Phase:

NET CARB COUNT:

Breakfast:

Lunch:

Dinner:

Snacks:

Beverages:

TOTAL DAILY NET CARBS:

Supplements taken:

Water Intake:

Exercise:

Day 94

Today's date is:

NET CARB LEVEL:

Phase:

NET CARB COUNT:

Breakfast:

Lunch:

Dinner:

Snacks:

Beverages:

TOTAL DAILY NET CARBS:

Supplements taken:

Water Intake:

Exercise:

Day 95

Today's date is:

NET CARB LEVEL: ( )

Phase:

NET CARB COUNT:

Breakfast:

Lunch:

Dinner:

Snacks:

Beverages:

TOTAL DAILY NET CARBS: ( )

Supplements taken:

Water Intake:

Exercise:

Day 96

Today's date is:

NET CARB LEVEL: ⬭

Phase:

NET CARB
COUNT:

Breakfast:

Lunch:

Dinner:

Snacks:

Beverages:

TOTAL DAILY NET CARBS: ⬭

Supplements taken:

Water Intake:

Exercise:

Day 97

NET CARB LEVEL:

Phase:

NET CARB COUNT:

Breakfast:

Lunch:

Dinner:

Snacks:

Beverages:

TOTAL DAILY NET CARBS:

Supplements taken:

Water Intake:

Exercise:

Day 98

NET CARB LEVEL:

Phase:

NET CARB COUNT:

Breakfast:

Lunch:

Dinner:

Snacks:

Beverages:

TOTAL DAILY NET CARBS:

Supplements taken:

Water Intake:

Exercise:

Week 14

TAKING STOCK

Weight

Measurements

BUST/CHEST:

WAIST:

HIPS:

UPPER ARMS:

THIGHS:

Rate the Following

Sticking to the programme
- ❏ excellent
- ❏ good
- ❏ need help

Exercise
- ❏ daily
- ❏ 1–3x/week
- ❏ nonexistent

Taking supplements
- ❏ always
- ❏ sometimes
- ❏ never

Mood
- ❏ positive
- ❏ neutral
- ❏ negative

Energy
- ❏ high
- ❏ medium
- ❏ low

Did you have cravings this week? Did you try to resist them? Were you successful?

What other challenges did you face this week?

Were you able to overcome them? If so, how? If not, what might help you do so?

Did you face any stressful situations? How did they affect your adherence to the programme?

What new foods/recipes did you add this week?

What is working for you? What changes do you need to make?

Week

15

Day 99

NET CARB LEVEL:

Phase:

NET CARB
COUNT:

Breakfast:

Lunch:

Dinner:

Snacks:

Beverages:

TOTAL DAILY NET CARBS:

Supplements taken:

Water Intake:

Exercise:

Day 100

Today's date is:

NET CARB LEVEL:

Phase:

NET CARB
COUNT:

Breakfast:

Lunch:

Dinner:

Snacks:

Beverages:

TOTAL DAILY NET CARBS:

Supplements taken:

Water Intake:

Exercise:

Day 101

NET CARB LEVEL:

Phase:

NET CARB COUNT:

Breakfast:

Lunch:

Dinner:

Snacks:

Beverages:

TOTAL DAILY NET CARBS:

Supplements taken:

Water Intake:

Exercise:

Day 102

NET CARB LEVEL:

Phase:

NET CARB COUNT:

Breakfast:

Lunch:

Dinner:

Snacks:

Beverages:

TOTAL DAILY NET CARBS:

Supplements taken:

Water Intake:

Exercise:

Day 103

Today's date is:

NET CARB LEVEL:

Phase:

NET CARB COUNT:

Breakfast:

Lunch:

Dinner:

Snacks:

Beverages:

TOTAL DAILY NET CARBS:

Supplements taken:

Water Intake:

Exercise:

Day 104

NET CARB LEVEL:

Phase:

NET CARB COUNT:

Breakfast:

Lunch:

Dinner:

Snacks:

Beverages:

TOTAL DAILY NET CARBS:

Supplements taken:

Water Intake:

Exercise:

Day 105

NET CARB LEVEL:

Phase:

NET CARB COUNT:

Breakfast:

Lunch:

Dinner:

Snacks:

Beverages:

TOTAL DAILY NET CARBS:

Supplements taken:

Water Intake:

Exercise:

Week 15

TAKING STOCK

Weight

Measurements

BUST/CHEST:

WAIST:

HIPS:

UPPER ARMS:

THIGHS:

Rate the Following

Sticking to the programme
- ❏ excellent
- ❏ good
- ❏ need help

Exercise
- ❏ daily
- ❏ 1–3x/week
- ❏ nonexistent

Taking supplements
- ❏ always
- ❏ sometimes
- ❏ never

Mood
- ❏ positive
- ❏ neutral
- ❏ negative

Energy
- ❏ high
- ❏ medium
- ❏ low

Did you have cravings this week? Did you try to resist them? Were you successful?

What other challenges did you face this week?

Were you able to overcome them? If so, how? If not, what might help you do so?

Did you face any stressful situations? How did they affect your adherence to the programme?

What new foods/recipes did you add this week?

What is working for you? What changes do you need to make?

Week 16

Day 106

Today's date is:

NET CARB LEVEL:

Phase:

NET CARB
COUNT:

Breakfast:

Lunch:

Dinner:

Snacks:

Beverages:

TOTAL DAILY NET CARBS:

Supplements taken:

Water Intake:

Exercise:

Day 107

NET CARB LEVEL:

Phase:

NET CARB COUNT:

Breakfast:

Lunch:

Dinner:

Snacks:

Beverages:

TOTAL DAILY NET CARBS:

Supplements taken:

Water Intake:

Exercise:

Day 108

NET CARB LEVEL:

Phase:

NET CARB
COUNT:

Breakfast:

Lunch:

Dinner:

Snacks:

Beverages:

TOTAL DAILY NET CARBS:

Supplements taken:

Water Intake:

Exercise:

Day 109

NET CARB LEVEL:

Phase:

NET CARB COUNT:

Breakfast:

Lunch:

Dinner:

Snacks:

Beverages:

TOTAL DAILY NET CARBS:

Supplements taken:

Water Intake:

Exercise:

Day 110

NET CARB LEVEL:

Phase:

NET CARB COUNT:

Breakfast:

Lunch:

Dinner:

Snacks:

Beverages:

TOTAL DAILY NET CARBS:

Supplements taken:

Water Intake:

Exercise:

Day 111

NET CARB LEVEL:

Phase:

NET CARB
COUNT:

Breakfast:

Lunch:

Dinner:

Snacks:

Beverages:

TOTAL DAILY NET CARBS:

Supplements taken:

Water Intake:

Exercise:

Day 112

Today's date is:

NET CARB LEVEL:

Phase:

NET CARB
COUNT:

Breakfast:

Lunch:

Dinner:

Snacks:

Beverages:

TOTAL DAILY NET CARBS:

Supplements taken:

Water Intake:

Exercise:

Week 16

TAKING STOCK

Weight

Measurements

BUST/CHEST:

WAIST:

HIPS:

UPPER ARMS:

THIGHS:

Rate the Following

Sticking to the programme
- ❏ excellent
- ❏ good
- ❏ need help

Exercise
- ❏ daily
- ❏ 1–3x/week
- ❏ nonexistent

Taking supplements
- ❏ always
- ❏ sometimes
- ❏ never

Mood
- ❏ positive
- ❏ neutral
- ❏ negative

Energy
- ❏ high
- ❏ medium
- ❏ low

Did you have cravings this week? Did you try to resist them? Were you successful?

What other challenges did you face this week?

Were you able to overcome them? If so, how? If not, what might help you do so?

Did you face any stressful situations? How did they affect your adherence to the programme?

What new foods/recipes did you add this week?

What is working for you? What changes do you need to make?

Week

17

Day 113

NET CARB LEVEL:

Phase:

NET CARB COUNT:

Breakfast:

Lunch:

Dinner:

Snacks:

Beverages:

TOTAL DAILY NET CARBS:

Supplements taken:

Water Intake:

Exercise:

Day 114

NET CARB LEVEL:

Phase:

NET CARB COUNT:

Breakfast:

Lunch:

Dinner:

Snacks:

Beverages:

TOTAL DAILY NET CARBS:

Supplements taken:

Water Intake:

Exercise:

Day 115

Today's date is:

NET CARB LEVEL: ◯

Phase:

NET CARB COUNT:

Breakfast:

Lunch:

Dinner:

Snacks:

Beverages:

TOTAL DAILY NET CARBS: ◯

Supplements taken:

Water Intake:

Exercise:

Day 116

NET CARB LEVEL: ⬭

Phase:

NET CARB COUNT:

Breakfast:

Lunch:

Dinner:

Snacks:

Beverages:

TOTAL DAILY NET CARBS: ⬭

Supplements taken:

Water Intake:

Exercise:

Day 117

NET CARB LEVEL:

Phase:

NET CARB COUNT:

Breakfast:

Lunch:

Dinner:

Snacks:

Beverages:

TOTAL DAILY NET CARBS:

Supplements taken:

Water Intake:

Exercise:

Day 118

NET CARB LEVEL:

Phase:

NET CARB COUNT:

Breakfast:

Lunch:

Dinner:

Snacks:

Beverages:

TOTAL DAILY NET CARBS:

Supplements taken:

Water Intake:

Exercise:

Day 119

NET CARB LEVEL: ⬭

Phase:

NET CARB COUNT:

Breakfast:

Lunch:

Dinner:

Snacks:

Beverages:

TOTAL DAILY NET CARBS: ⬭

Supplements taken:

Water Intake:

Exercise:

Week 17

TAKING STOCK

Weight

Measurements

BUST/CHEST:

WAIST:

HIPS:

UPPER ARMS:

THIGHS:

Rate the Following

Sticking to the programme
- ❏ excellent
- ❏ good
- ❏ need help

Exercise
- ❏ daily
- ❏ 1–3x/week
- ❏ nonexistent

Taking supplements
- ❏ always
- ❏ sometimes
- ❏ never

Mood
- ❏ positive
- ❏ neutral
- ❏ negative

Energy
- ❏ high
- ❏ medium
- ❏ low

Did you have cravings this week? Did you try to resist them? Were you successful?

What other challenges did you face this week?

Were you able to overcome them? If so, how? If not, what might help you do so?

Did you face any stressful situations? How did they affect your adherence to the programme?

What new foods/recipes did you add this week?

What is working for you? What changes do you need to make?

Day 120

Today's date is:

NET CARB LEVEL:

Phase:

NET CARB COUNT:

Breakfast:

Lunch:

Dinner:

Snacks:

Beverages:

TOTAL DAILY NET CARBS:

Supplements taken:

Water Intake:

Exercise:

Fibre: A Special Kind of Carbohydrate

Dietary fibre is the indigestible parts of plant cells. Although it is a carbohydrate, fibre does not convert to glucose and thus does not raise your blood-sugar level the way carbohydrates typically do.

In fact, fibre actually slows the entry of glucose into the bloodstream. This, in turn, reduces the blood-sugar spikes that cause insulin production and encourage the body to produce and store body fat. And by slowing down the transit time of foods in the digestive tract, fibre helps you feel full longer, resulting in fewer food cravings. Fibre also:

- Binds to cholesterol in the intestine, helping rid the body of it
- Absorbs and then eliminates bacterial toxins in the intestine
- Reduces the likelihood of getting diverticulitis
- Speeds the excretion of gallstone-promoting bile
- Supports the immune system by crowding out harmful bacteria in the colon
- Bulks up the stool and make it easier to pass

Fibre-rich foods include vegetables, nuts and seeds, fruit, beans and whole unrefined grains. During Induction your primary source of fibre will be vegetables. (In later phases you introduce other sources of fibre.) You can get the benefits of fibre without the carbs contained in these foods by supplementing your diet with as a tablespoon or two of psyllium husks daily. Be sure to select a sugar-free product. You can also use coarse wheat bran or flaxseed meal. Although it's derived from grain, coarse bran is pure fiber so it doesn't add to your carb count. Mix Psyllium husks with water, or you can sprinkle bran over your vegetables, or blend flaxseed meal into a shake. Drinking the recommended eight glasses or more of water daily is also essential to avoid constipation. Also remember that you need to accompany any increase in fibre intake with plenty of water.

Consuming too much fibre can block mineral absorption because food simply doesn't stay in the digestive tract long enough for your body to extract valuable nutrients. Gas, flatulence or constipation can also result. If you haven't been eating significant amounts of fibre, increase your intake gradually to allow the intestinal tract to adjust.

The Importance of Water

On any eating regime, a minimum of 1.8 litres/64 fl oz, or eight 225-ml/8-fl oz glasses, of water per day is the usual recommendation. Many people, particularly women, suffer from inadequate hydration, so it is important to be diligent about drinking water throughout the day. Water consumption will also help to flush toxins from your body and combat such problems as constipation and bad breath. Note that coffee, tea and diet fizzy drinks do not apply to the daily minimum, but are over and above it.

Eating on the Road

There is no question that travel can make it harder to stay with any weight-management programme. The key to staying on track is a combination of mental and physical preparation. The following tips should help ensure that you don't leave your progress behind when you're on the road.

- **Think 'big picture'.** Don't use your trip as an excuse to go off the programme. Remember, if you continually take detours from your planned route, you'll never reach your destination.

- **Take it with you.** Pack some low carb snack foods, such as 25-g/1-oz portions of cheese wrapped in cling film. If you're travelling by car, pack a cool bag with cold cuts and cheese or salad. Or stow away a few Atkins bars and some shake mix to use as meal replacements.

- **Eat first.** Start out on the right foot by eating a well-planned, satisfying meal before you set out on your trip.

- **Go a little nuts.** Snack on nuts and seeds, which are high in protein and fat. You'll feel more satisfied and in control of your appetite after eating a handful. Go easy on these snack options if you are in the Induction phase, particularly if you find it difficult to lose weight.

- **Don't skip meals.** Omitting a meal could make you ravenous, out of control, and more likely to grab anything edible.

- **Fly right.** If you're on a flight where a meal will be served, call ahead and ask what's on the menu. You can probably find a seafood or chicken salad or another dish you can rework.

- **Drink up.** Consume lots of water, which will help you feel satisfyingly full. But stay away from coffee and diet drinks full of caffeine, which may increase carbohydrate cravings.

- **Pack your pills.** Once one element of your routine gets upset, other good habits tend to slide as well. Even if you make some mistakes with your food choices, staying on your supplements will help you focus on getting back to eating properly.

- **Speed counts.** If you do slip off the programme for a day or more, get back on ASAP. The longer you're derailed, the harder it may be to get back on track.

Don't Even Go There

If you find all your food options on the road are poor, adhere to the programme as closely as you can. For example, eat more salad and other vegetables than your usual allowance. That doesn't mean that you might as well eat bread and pasta. It's better to deviate a little than to toss the whole programme out the window.

Finally, remember who's boss. You are in control of what goes in your mouth at all times – even when you're not in your own home. When dining out, ask how things are prepared and give instructions. After all, you're paying for it. Even in a fast-food restaurant, you're entitled to 'have it your way'. Why should some stranger determine the success of your programme – or your health?

Make Fast Food Friendly

Sandwich shops: Chicken or tuna salad is a good choice. Alternatively, ask for turkey, roast beef, cheese and sausage, but try to steer clear of salami and other meat products preserved with nitrates. Ask for your selection on a plate instead of on a roll, and you're ready to rock.

Burger chains: Sandwiches are usually a good bet. Just toss the bun. Mayo and mustard are permissible but beware of ketchup, which often contains a lot of sugar. Watch out, too, for special sauces, as they also often have sugar in them. Tomato slices and lettuce are fine. Steer clear of anything advertised as 'low-fat', a label that often translates to high carb.

Fried chicken places: Avoid anything barbecued or breaded. Barbecue sauce is typically full of sugar and even if you remove the skin, the sugar has probably seeped into the meat. Dry-rubbed meats are fine, as are roasted chicken and side dishes such as a tossed salad. If there's a grilled chicken fillet sandwich available, grab it! Discard the bun, and you've got a pretty good selection. Or scrape the breading off a fried chicken breast.

Salad bars: Here you'll find the choices you need for a nutritious meal. Use olive oil and regular red- or white-wine vinegar instead of a prepared dressing; commercial dressings and balsamic vinegars often contain sugar. Baked stuffed potatoes are an absolute no-no.

Unless you're starving, avoid fast food, Mexican-style and pizza restaurants, ice cream shops and bakeries.

PLACE YOUR
PHOTO HERE

This is me after doing Atkins